# After My Brain Broke

# (My Story Of Loss And Discovery Of Secrets)

By

Global-Award Winning Corporate Mental Health Facilitator, Burnout Prevention Educator and Burnout Hacker

Laurence Nicholson of burnout-hacker.com

2021 - burnout-hacker.com Rights Reserved

## FOREWORD...

This book represents both a warning of what can happen due to stress, especially from the workplace, and a set of 'Hacks', that took me a number of years of research and testing to develop, for avoiding the traumas described.

If you just want to find out the secret hacks I developed, then just go straight to the section 'The Development Of Hacks', but if you are interested in WHY I ended up needing them, and the extent to which burnout trauma can impact your life, I recommend reading my story from the beginning!

In the ebook, the 'Hacks' are shown in red, and for quick reference (and for the paperback/hardback), there is a summary of the 'Hacks' included and the sections they can be found in, at the end of the book.

Where reference is made to my **Cognitive Masterclass**, more information can be found at https://burnout-hacker.com

Cover Photo 109489906 © Teodoro Ortiz Tarrascusa | Dreamstime.com

# Part One

## Before The Break!

## *All Good Here...*

**1988**

After a few years exploring opportunities in our prestigious Foreign & Commonwealth Office and the Ministry Of Defence, I realised I was not going to find the challenges I craved within that sector and I stepped out of that world into one of 'looking for my next role'.

There were no on-line agencies, digital job marketplaces, LinkedIn, Indeed or other job boards, back then, (Even 'Monster' had not been created then), so I headed into my local high street temp agency shop, and basically said "have you any jobs available?"

I think I expected them to say "Sure. Choose from one of these" as they handed me a list of jobs available, as I was relatively naive back then with regard the private sector. Obviously, that scenario did not happen.

What DID happen was the recruitment consultant asked me what I was looking for and what qualifications I had..............and my day sank into an emptiness.

After a long conversation, I had arrived at a professional qualification I would register for, and a basic temporary role with a local company I would be interviewed for, to do whilst I was qualifying.

**1991**

Fast forward 3 years, and I was a newly qualified technical systems accountant, and I was about to start a role with a global oil company whose head office was just down the road, which would be the 'touch-paper' that lit my super successful career in corporate consulting.

**1992 - 2008 (The 'Flying High Years)**

During these year I established myself as a specialist in many functions working across corporate environments, as both a consultant and leader, and both worked and lived in scores of locations around the world. I became a renowned adviser and consultant in procurement, finance, law, information technology, organisational change and executive management, for many global organisations.

I lived a dream lifestyle, in a large house we'd had built, new top of the range top named cars, exotic holidays, and first class global travel.

I was flying high, and I was sure my purpose was to provide my expertise and knowledge to top 100 global corporates and C-Suite Executives, in return for ludicrous fees and bonuses, and top flight corporate style benefits.

I was turning down offers left and right, as I was so busy that, at one point, my availability was becoming 12+ months ahead!

I was dealing with massive pressures from starting up my own businesses, leading and advising for global named organisations, jet-setting around the globe, available and on call 24/7, all with apparent ease....I was 'indestructible'.

Or so I thought.

# Part Two
## How My Sky Fell In

## *The First Tremor...*

**2008**

It all seemed normal.

My week had been no more busy than usual, and I was a few days back from a 3 week global tour of leadership workshops, preparing for a weekend with my family, trying to clear all the urgent issues from my list.

It was a Thursday, and I was in the office early, as usual.

I had been in since 7am, and had prepared all my notes for the full day of meetings, made sure all the logistics had been taken care of, meeting rooms were ready and all the tech was working and connecting properly for those international attendees.

The first session was due to start at 1000, so I decided to get myself a coffee from the on-site shop, and relax for the 30 minutes or so I had before the start. It was London, June, and a pleasant but not overly hot day (standard London summer), and I was waiting in the queue for the Barista to ask for my order, feeling quite relaxed and ready for the day.

My turn came, and I looked up as I heard the "what can I get you?" and for about 5 seconds, but what seemed a lifetime, I could not think or even process the question. It was a very strange experience, and I theatrically shook my head, and 'came back to earth' and ordered my drink. I put it down to the traveling and too little sleep.

The first couple of meetings went well, and so they should what with the amount of planning and preparation I had put in.

The second session after lunch had started, and I was settling back after my introduction, to listen and critique the strategy suggestions the leadership were creating, when I went blank.

I could hear and see the people around me, even hear the question they were asking me and recognised the words, but I could not relate them to any form of understanding or context.

I had suffered a mental stall.

Unlike the 5 second experience I had had earlier, this failed to clear, and I had to be taken to the private hospital under the corporate health plan, and be assessed.

Things started to clear enough for me to grasp the gist of the words I was hearing, and understand I had suffered, what in those days was called, a 'nervous breakdown'. What we generally call a burnout today.

I had exhausted my cognitive capacity below an easily recoverable threshold.

I was admitted for a few days, given medications to shut down parts of my cognitive processing, and placed on a recovery plan which included being 'signed off' for a period of 6 MONTHS.

It took 10 days before I could communicate effectively, and somewhat 'normally', despite being painfully aware of the very worried looks on the faces of my family.

My recovery seemed to accelerate after that, and I was frankly feeling frustrated after about 9 weeks, and getting irritable about not being back at work, so I took the decision (and I take full responsibility for this) to return to work the start of the next month, which was a couple of weeks away. I actually had announced to my family I was going back immediately, but was 'negotiated' down to the next month.

It was heading towards Autumn and Winter, so I was thinking about my travel plans, looking to head to the warmer climes, and prioritised workshop and training requests from those in such places.

My return was a great success, and all my clients were very happy to see me 'back on my feet', and I spent pretty much all of the winter of 2008 and spring of 2009 overseas, back in the seat and as busy as ever.

I returned back to the UK in the Summer of 2009, to work with my European clients.

## The BIG One...

**2009**

Being back in the is always a wonderful feeling, especially after being away for a longer length of time, and this time was no exception.

I had had a great world tour' and been exceptionally busy, sometimes flying 'red-eye' from country to country, going straight into another set of workshops, just to get all my clients into my schedule.

My return to 'Blighty' was no different. Back to back client workshops and hopping all over the country, almost from the moment I landed back.

It was a beautiful, calm, sunny but cold November Wednesday, and I was sitting in the head office of a client in London, taking a final look over my materials for their workshop, which I was starting in 45 minutes at 1045.

I had been trying to shake a 'niggling' headache since the weekend, but generally just ignoring it as it was just a minor irritant in the back of my mind.

My Wife had asked me a few times, since my return if I was ok, saying I looked a bit 'washed out and tired', but I felt fine and said as much, going so far as to say I actually felt better than ever, and not to worry so much!

I checked my watch and ............ my world stopped!

I sat struggling to make any sense of what I was seeing, what I was hearing, and simply could not get ANY focus on any single thought. It was like trying to call to mind a dream, only for it to elude any attempt to get it to front of mind!

I struggled to even move, as my brain couldn't make any neural associations with simple tasks.

I guess it took some time for people to realise something was wrong, as I was just sitting staring strangely at my surroundings, and it was when I was not responding to any questions, that the panic button was hit.

All I saw was a lot of different people coming and going, speaking to me and with each other, but I could make no sense of what they were saying.

Once again I found myself in a medical centre, this time completely unable to get any grasp on what was happening.

Later I found out my 'tender' repairs in my brain from my previous breakdown, had failed and the processes in my brain were out of control. The 'attenuator' function of my selective attention circuit was triggering randomly and effectively preventing any thought from getting through the filtering process. (See ringed area of the Diagram of Treismon's Attenuation Theory, below)

This meant no thoughts or inputs were getting sufficient contextual attachments to be able to be processed in my pre-frontal cortex.

It is like entering a party and not being able to choose which group of people to go and talk to, but constantly trying to decide.

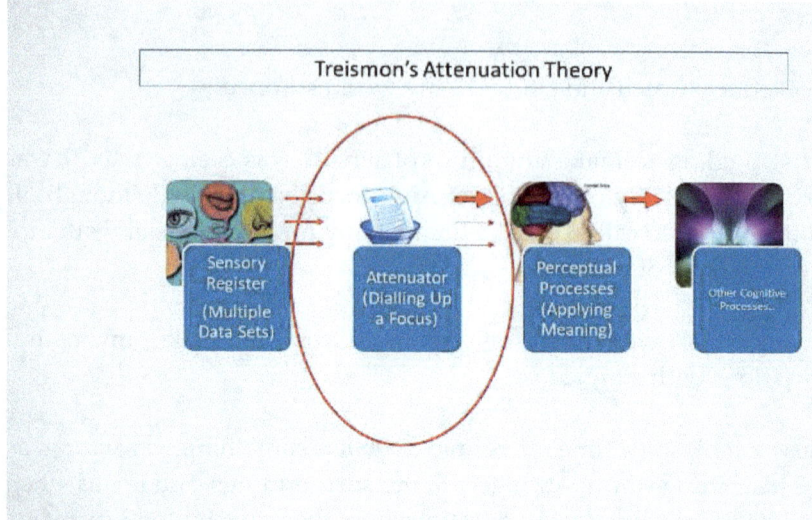

As predicted by a number of people, all of whom I had arrogantly ignored, I had returned far too soon, and my brain had effectively and spectacularly closed itself down to protect itself, after not being allowed to rebuild from the first trauma.

As my step-grandson called it: My Brain had Broken!

## *My World Collapses...*

It took nearly 3 months before anything started making any sense, and most of the time I was on medication which made me sleep.

I could see very worried faces, and feel the concern as almost a tangible atmosphere, and as I very slowly started getting some semblance of cognition and understanding back, the reality of the seriousness of this breakdown started to hit home.

Little did I know at that point, that that was literally going to happen.

I was unable to function.

I was unable to earn.

I was a burden to my family and friends.

We struggled on as a family for the first year, with my Wife having to find a job on top of looking after our family and me.

All I could do was look on, sometimes still having periods of relapse, when I would stare, not comprehending my surroundings, and watch my family struggle so much. I think I was the lucky one really, as much of the time I simply didn't understand enough to be able to feel the emotional trauma they were all going through.

The first to go were the cars.

As much as my family and friends could do, they could not generate anywhere near the income I was before, and cutback after cutback had to be made, creating a seemingly insurmountable level of pressure on those around me.

I remember wondering why the tow trucks were taking the cars of our driveway, but that fleeting thought soon disintegrated like the others and I shifted my gaze somewhere else.

Our regular holidays had also been forfeited, as well as expensive weekends, dinners and even school trips which had to be paid for.

All the while, even though I was slowly regaining some functioning, I was almost casually drifting around watching what felt unreal.

After 18 months, we (and I mean the family) sold the house. It was a big expense which they had desperately tried to hang on to, but in the end it became too much, and we drastically downsized. It would provide some respite from the pressure of bills for a couple of years, and was absolutely the right thing to do.

Around the 2 years mark, I had regained much of my cognitive performance, although I was very weak and my brain tired very easily and still struggled a lot with focus and any kind of creative thinking.

I thought it a miracle our family had managed to stay together, through all the trauma.

Sadly, even that would not survive the experience, and it broke apart a few years later.

All I knew from that year 2, when I was able to start any significant cognitive processing, was that I could not go through, nor put anyone else through, another burnout.

I HAD to learn how to prevent this happening!

# Part Three
## The Rebuild

## *The Research Years...*

Whenever I had prolonged lucid periods, and my focus was operating with some level of effectiveness, I started to throw myself into searching for any research I could find regarding the way our brains operate, how stress affects the various elements of our brain structures, and what we needed to understand in order to protect our cognitive performance and structure our cognitive workload appropriately.

What I found was years of research articles, experiments, theories and scholarly articles on the neuroscience of the brain, our psychology and how our thoughts and decisions are subject to heuristics and bias, and pattern storage theories, attenuation of focus theories and much MUCH more.

Experts and scientists were looking into every aspect of our brains, and much of what I discovered was incredible, enlightening, but also a little frustrating. Quite a lot I struggled to understand, partly because of my condition and partly because the science was alien to me and beyond my comprehension, but I carried on. I learnt. I searched. I cross referenced.

I was also frustrated because, despite all of the hundreds and hundreds of articles, papers, theses and results I trawled through, I found very little that I could directly apply.

It was about 6 month into the research, when I hit on a notion that I needed to look at this in a different way.

Looking back, I think it was one of the first truly creative cognitive efforts I experienced after the burnout, and it proved to be a pivotal moment for me.

I had been 'knee deep' in a number of studies on cognitive loading including the following, which I have included an abstract from:

### 1. Brain States: Top-Down Influences in Sensory Processing

> Charles D. Gilbert and Mariano Sigman
> The Rockefeller University

**ABSTRACT:** *All cortical and thalamic levels of sensory processing are subject to powerful top-down influences, the shaping of lower-level processes by more complex information. New findings on the diversity of top-down interactions show that cortical areas function as adaptive processors, being subject to attention, expectation, and perceptual task. Brain states are determined by the interactions between multiple cortical areas and the modulation of intrinsic circuits by feedback connections. In perceptual learning, both the encoding and recall of learned information involves a selection of the appropriate inputs that convey information about the stimulus being discriminated. Disruption of this interaction may lead to behavioural disorders, including schizophrenia.*

### 2. PAUSES AS INDICATORS OF COGNITIVE EFFORT IN POST-EDITING MACHINE TRANSLATION OUTPUT.

SHARON O'BRIEN
School of Applied Language and Intercultural Studies, Dublin City University

**ABSTRACT:** In translation process and language production research, pauses are seen as indicators of cognitive processing. Investigating the correlations between source text machine translatability and post-editing effort involves an assessment of cognitive effort. Therefore, an analysis of pauses is essential. This paper presents data from a research project which includes an analysis of pauses in post-editing, triangulated with the Choice Network Analysis method and Translog. Results suggest that the pause-to-keyboarding ratio does not differ significantly for sentences deemed to be more suitable for machine translation than for those deemed to be less suitable. Also, results confirm the finding in research elsewhere that pause duration and frequency is subject to individual differences. Finally, we suggest that while pauses provide some indication of cognitive processing, supplementary methods are required to give a fuller picture.

## 3. Different effects of pausing on cognitive load in a medical simulation game

Joy Yeonjoo Lee, Jeroen J.G. van Merrienboera, Jeroen Donkers, Halszka Jarodzka, Geraldine Sellenraad
School of Health Professions Education, Maastricht University, P.O. Box 616, 6200 MD Maastricht, the Netherlands

*Welten Institute, Open University of The Netherlands, PO Box 2960, 6401 DL Heerlen, the Netherlands*

*Faculty of Health, Medicine and Life Sciences, Maastricht University, P.O. Box 616, 6200 MD Maastricht, the Netherlands*

**ABSTRACT:** *In medical training, allowing learners to take pauses during tasks is known to enhance performance. Cognitive load theory assumes that insertion of pauses positively affects cognitive load, thereby enhancing performance. However, empirical studies on how allowing and taking pauses affects cognitive load and performance in dynamic task environments are scarce. We investigated the pause effect, using a computerised simulation game in emergency medicine. Medical students (N = 70) were randomly assigned to one of two conditions: simulation with (n = 40) and without (n = 30) the option to take pauses. All participants played the same two scenarios, during which game logs and eye-tracking data were recorded. Overall, both cognitive load and performance were higher in the condition with pauses than in the one without. The act of pausing, however, temporarily lowered cognitive load, especially during intense moments. Two different manifestations of the pause effect were identified: (1) by stimulating additional cognitive and meta-cognitive processes, pauses increased overall cognitive load; and (2) through relaxation, the act of pausing temporarily decreased heightened cognitive load. Consequently, our results suggest that in* order to enhance students' performance and learning it is important that we encourage them to utilise the different effects of pausing.

## 4. Pausing Strategies as Means of Information Processing in Spontaneous Narratives

Miguel Oliveira
  Instituto de Lingüística Teórica e Computacional (ILTEC) Lisbon, Portugal

**ABSTRACT:** This paper investigates the role of pause in the process of information organisation in narrative discourse. Following the cognitive research on pausing strategies, the present study assumes that the frequency of pause usage varies as a function of the content of the individual sections in a narrative. The material used for the analysis consisted of a number of spontaneous narratives. The results failed to demonstrate any association between type of information and pausing phenomena, but it revealed the existence of a pattern of varying hesitancy that generally correspond to the different sections in a narrative. This would suggest that pausing in narrative is primarily governed by the cognitive rhythm of speech.

## 5. Disturbing the rhythm of thought: Speech pausing patterns in schizophrenia, with and without formal thought disorder.

Derya Cokal 1*, Vitor Zimmerer 2*, Douglas Turkington 3*4*, Nicol Ferrier 3*4*, Rosemary Varley 2*, Stuart Watson 3*4*,

Wolfram Hinzen 5*6*7*

1* School of Engineering and Computer Science, Queen Mary University of London
2* Department of Language and Cognition, University College London
3* Institute of Neuroscience, Newcastle University
4* Northumberland Tyne and Wear NHS Foundation Trust
5* ICREA (Institucio´ Catalana de Recerca i Estudis Avanc.ats), Barcelona
6* Department of Translation and Language Sciences, Universitat Pompeu Fabra, Barcelona
7* FIDMAG Germanes Hospitalaries Research Foundation, Benito Menni Hospital, Barcelona

**ABSTRACT:** Everyday speech is produced with an intricate timing pattern and rhythm. Speech units follow each other with short interleaving pauses, which can be either bridged by fillers (erm, ah) or empty. Through their syntactic positions, pauses connect to the thoughts expressed. We investigated whether disturbances of thought in schizophrenia are manifest in patterns at this level of linguistic organisation, whether these are seen in first degree relatives (FDR) and how specific they are to formal thought disorder (FTD). Spontaneous speech from 15 participants without FTD (SZ-FTD), 15 with FTD (SZ+FTD), 15 FDRs and 15 neurotypical controls (NC) was obtained from a comic strip retelling task and rated for pauses sub-classified by syntactic position and duration. SZ-FTD produced significantly more unfilled pauses than NC in utterance-

> *initial positions and before embedded clauses. Unfilled pauses occur- ring within clausal units did not distinguish any groups. SZ-FTD also differed from SZ+FTD in producing significantly more pauses before embedded clauses. SZ+FTD differed from NC and FDR only in producing longer utterance-initial pauses. FDRs produced significantly fewer fillers than NC. Results reveal that the temporal organisation of speech is an important window on disturbances of the thought process and how these relate to language.*

What became clear, was that the vast majority of the research on cognitive load in which 'identified cognitive reactions and effects' had been noticed, went on to focus on why this happened and what the trigger was. Almost none of it considered what benefits could be derived from 'deliberately' applying such 'reactions' under everyday, and subsequently stressful, situations.

It was in the work "Different effects of pausing on cognitive load in a medical simulation game" (#3 above), that I noticed the elements which grabbed my attention (pun intended!) referencing the effects of pausing on cognitive load. I specifically picked up on the following extracts, highlighted:

> ==*The act of pausing, however, temporarily lowered cognitive load, especially during intense moments*==. *Two different manifestations of the pause effect were identified: (1) by stimulating additional cognitive and meta-cognitive processes, pauses increased overall cognitive load; and (2)* ==*through relaxation, the act of pausing temporarily decreased heightened cognitive load*==. *Consequently, our results suggest that in order to enhance students' performance and learning it is important that we encourage them to* ==*utilise the different effects of pausing.*==

This kicked off a process in my recovering mind, which went on to form the basis for one of my most successful 'hacks', that of **Thought Transfer** or **Thought Pausing.**

## *Testing, Testing...*

I was getting stronger, mentally, every day, and I believe the effort I was putting into my research was helping that process, because it was working my brain (kind of exercise if you like) but without any significant level of stress, as my family was still shielding me from that!

This gave my brain free rein to get abstract in its thinking, and approach things from new directions, and I started looking into all the ways I could think of, to take advantage of the protective tricks the brain applies to deal with pressures and stresses it encounters all the time.

I spent almost 9 months trimming down lists, removing research which had mediocre results or only worked for a small sample group, and fine tuning my own approaches to these, in order to get to a small set of around 3 or 4 'hacks' or cognitive techniques for a set of what I considered the most prevalent issues faced both at work and outside of work.

Now I had to find out which were the most effective, across the widest range of test subjects as possible. This required testing groups with various cultural and behavioural characteristics, and so I put together a set of what I called 'exploratory workshops', where I taught a number of different collections of techniques, like a multiple A-B test, in order to get to a single optimum 'hack' for each subject area relating to the most prevalent issues I identified earlier.

What you will read about in the next Chapter, are the absolute best hacks identified for each of the categories, and which form the basis of my global training courses, for which I was honoured in a 2021 global award by Brainz Magazine.

# Part Four

## The Development Of Hacks

## *The Brain & Intelligence...*

I think we all know that there is a lot of 'noise' in the world we live in these days, from conversations to arguments, emails to phone calls, and TV to radio, and our brains create their own in the form of self talk (thoughts), both positive and negative.

In fact, research has estimated we typically have some 50,000 thoughts EVERY DAY, and this only increases as the amount of interference and distraction increases.

Now our brains are incredible and, to be honest, unfathomable in how they actually operate on an existential level, and clearly getting busier by the day, but they are also fragile.

As a structure, our brains are quite mind-blowing, each one having Approximately 80 billion nerve cells, called neurons. Eighty billion (80,000,000,000)! That is more than 10 times as many neurons in each brain as there are people living on Earth

A single neuron may contain thousands of synapses, which are that small pocket of space between two cells where they can pass messages to communicate.

In fact, one type of neuron called the Purkinje cell, found in the brain's cerebellum, is thought to have as many as one hundred thousand synapses, and there are approximately 125 trillion synapses, just in the cerebral cortex alone, That's roughly equal to the number of stars in 1,500 Milky Way Galaxies!

With this in mind (excuse THIS pun!), it is really not surprising that our brains get tired quickly, and is most often the weakest link in our performance.

We do, however have critical parts of our brains which have significantly limited resources. Resources it burns through very quickly, and because we have limited mental resources, it is important to understand how our brain works, so that we can know how to help ease the burden!

That way, we can be better placed to make better decisions, which are then less costly than poorly formed, reactive ones, to both ourselves and our employers or own businesses!

It is well known through scientific study, that we have differing hemispheres to our brains, known as 'Brain Lateralisation', each hemisphere carrying out different controlling processes and applying different perspectives such as logical vs creative.

There is also a significant difference to the amount of knowledge or information, each area can hold and process.

When compared, if the system 2 pre-frontal cortex can hold, say 256 GB (an iPhone 8), then the system 1 Limbic system can hold 2,500,000 GB (2.5 PB). To put that in perspective, 2.5 PB is the amount of storage it would take for you to record 10,000 digital photos every day for your entire life!

Having discovered just how busy the mind is, and that there are numerous dimensions to it, around 'systems', hemispheres, scale of capacity differences between the limbic and pre-frontal cortex systems (all of which are covered in a great deal of detail in my Cognitive Masterclass), there emerged not only limitations, but also an age based degeneration in one of the two types of intelligence our brains hold.

When we are young, and are operating as the information sponges all children are, we are increasing the crystallised intelligence we store away, or the 'learned and experienced' knowledge.

This enters the large capacity limbic system (the 2.5 PB storage area) and is our store of knowledge we draw upon all through our lives. It holds much of the automatic pilot knowledge like how to drive a car or ride a bicycle, for instance.

Our other type of intelligence, our 'Fluid' intelligence, represents our ability to 'consider' our immediate surroundings and situation, and apply relevant and pertinent situational information, against previously learned and experienced knowledge, to determine the optimum solution for any current problem.

All this sounds great so far, right?

Unfortunately, our ability to hold on to these types of intelligence declines as we age, and not at the same rate.

As we age, our storage of new information flattens out after around 35 to 40, and degrades once we are heading past 60 to 65. This is not a huge issue, as it means we keep much of what we learn over our lifetime, as crystallised intelligence.

The PROBLEM is that our 'Fluid' intelligence, that part which allows us to apply the crystallised intelligence effectively and productively to issues or problems in the present moment, tends to peak around our 20's and begins to decline, increasing its rate at around the age of 40, on average.

There is some good news though, in the form of the cognitive HACK:

**Continued 'exercising' of what Hercule Poirot called the 'little grey cells', across the appropriate cognitive skills, can delay the onset of decline and reduce the gradient and ultimate intersection point of the crystallised and fluid intelligence gradients.**

There are many 'brain-training' resources available, and selecting those which have the most effective exercises, can have a beneficial effect, as long as they become part of everyday routines.

A more detailed explanation of which exercises are most effective is included in my Cognitive Masterclass training - See https://burnout-hacker.com.

## *Impulse Control...*

So what is 'Impulse Control'?

Basically, it is the exercise of constraint from automatic, emotive reaction or immediate gratification.

Self-control of your emotions affects your Impulse control, and therefor your decision making, because reactive behaviour results in rapid unconsidered decisions, which are rarely the most effective or productive.

Impulse control is managed within the pre-frontal cortex, and is a result of the chemical reaction between the synapses which triggers the electrical signals between the cells in the brain, so the problem is that we know that effort in the Pre-frontal Cortex can lead quickly to 'mental fatigue', because we know that this part of our brain is very resource hungry, and burns through energy quickly.

What do I mean by 'Mental Fatigue'?

Marcora et al. (2009) define mental fatigue as "a psychobiological state which is caused by prolonged periods of demanding cognitive activity."

When researching sports coaching, Hagger et al. (2010a, p. 67) in an article, came to the conclusion that "mental fatigue is analogous to ego depletion which relates to the area of physical performance, and likely coincides with the depletion of self-control", so it became clear that the world of sports performance can teach us about Impulse Control, and benefit us in other parts of life.

In order to understand and thus exercise our impulse control, it is important to apply conditions which require us to focus our attention on our impulsive reactions. This way, we create a neural association of our doing so (our self-control strength or Impulse-control strength), for us to draw upon when needed. In my Cognitive Masterclass Training, I go into detail about two particular types of exercise which create the perfect conditions.

Managing your impulse control often involves the concept of 'delayed gratification'. In a classic psychology experiment from the 1970s, a psychologist named Walter Mischel placed a sweet in front of children and offered them a choice. They could either enjoy the sweet now, or wait a brief period of time in order to get two sweets.

When the experimenter left the room, many of the children immediately ate the sweet, but some of them were able to put off the urge to enjoy the sweet now, and wait for the reward of getting two delicious goodies later on.

What Mischel discovered, was that those who were able to delay gratification, had a number of advantages later on, over those who simply could not wait.

The children who had waited for the sweet, were found to have performed better academically, years later.

Those who delayed their gratification, also displayed fewer behavioural problems and had better **current** school test scores.

Researchers have found that this ability to delay gratification, is not just an important part of goal achievement, but seems also to have a major impact on long-term life success and overall well-being.

One of the best 'hacks' for exercising and improving our impulse control, is the Stroop Test (explained in detail in my Cognitive Masterclass), and one many people are probably already familiar with, where words describing colours (red, blue, green, etc.) are flashed either on cards or on screen, but with the font also displayed in a colour, which might be different to the colour the word is describing, for example the word RED might be shown but displayed in BLUE ink/screen colour.

The exercise is to click a certain button or call out the colour of either the actual font colour OR the colour the word is describing.

This forces you to control the impulse to react immediately, and consider what you are seeing before you respond, which gets harder the longer you carry on the exercise, and much like physical exercise, builds stronger control over your impulse to react immediately.

There are problems with delaying gratification, and part of this is the perceived amount of time delay between the decision to delay, and the reward! The longer the time gap, the harder it is to choose to delay. (More problems and their identified solutions can be found in my Masterclass)

## *Attention...*

Hey, attention is relatively simple, right?

You are either 'present' or you are not, surely?

Actually No!

Remember when we talked about our brains 'systems' earlier?

The huge 25 PB engine of our limbic system, and its rapid speed. The energy hungry pre-frontal cortex, with its 215 GB of capacity, and slow high effort processing?

Well.... Attention is the 'Sweet Spot' between the two, where we maximise the use of the available knowledge (Crystallised Intelligence) with the application of minimal but necessary and intensely focused 'current situation' information (Fluid Intelligence).

It will come therefor as no surprise that attention is:

1 - Highly demanding of energy, and

2 - Fragile, easily broken through distraction.

So why do we need to be 'present'? What is so special about that?

Actually, we need to be 'present in the moment' for a number of reasons…

*We need to optimise meeting performance relating to decision making.*

*Everyone needs to be able to process and understand ALL the information available to the team.*

*This means using our pre-frontal cortex to pay attention to all the current situation information, and apply this to stored knowledge and understanding.*

*To do this we need to be truly present, listening and processing!*

There is obviously a short amount of time this is possible for before we lose focus and our limbic system starts taking control, as the regulating influence of the pre-frontal cortex fades under fatigue.

What does this mean for my work life? It means you need to structure your day appropriately, and optimise activities around how your brain works, such as making meetings brief, focused and with a highly attentive set of participants, who are NOT distracted.

So how can I be attentive if there are so many things competing for my focus, I hear you ask! (I know, because I asked this too way back when I was recovering)

Also, isn't this is the opposite of multitasking, (which of course is not actually possible. Rapid task switching is as near as you can get) that managers seem to expect these days?

YES! This is the ultimate 'Single-tasking' activity!. Focusing on one thing only.

It is possible, and very productive, but be aware though, that is has been proven to take an average of 25 minutes to regain focus after distraction, so if you need to focus on one critical issue, make sure you have dealt with or removed all distractions.

So, a 'quick check of email/facebook/LinkedIn' is in fact the 30 second 'quick check' PLUS up to 25 minutes to regain full focus!

**How can you 'hack' your brain and create an environment to assist in improving your ability to focus your attention?**

**Exercises! Focus exercises!**

**There are methods which make you focus and ignore external distractions, such as memory 'journey' exercises, which force you to spend longer focusing on remembering a set of steps, which in turn improves both your recall from working memory and your ability to 'zone out' local distractions.**

Look into taking my Masterclass, as we cover this in more detail, and practice the best methods which accelerate your selective attention abilities.

*Pauses, Peak Performance & Arousal Control...*

Pauses, are an interesting subject area, and have been studied for a long time now, but more typically on the basis of why they exist in certain people's behaviours.

I have already mentioned in the section "The Research Years", a number of research articles which looked into the 'phenomenon' of pausing, either in speech and linguistic patterns, or in cognitive behaviours under certain conditions.

I also indicated one of the reports that first made me think about pausing in a different way, which I have reproduced for you here:

```
3. Different effects of pausing on cognitive
load in a medical simulation game

Joy     Yeonjoo    Lee,    Jeroen    J.G.    van
Merrienboera,    Jeroen    Donkers,    Halszka
Jarodzka, Geraldine Sellenraad
   School of Health Professions Education,
Maastricht University, P.O. Box 616, 6200 MD
Maastricht, the Netherlands
   Welten Institute, Open University of The
Netherlands, PO Box 2960, 6401 DL Heerlen,
the Netherlands
   Faculty of Health, Medicine and Life
```

Sciences, Maastricht University, P.O. Box 616, 6200 MD Maastricht, the Netherlands

ABSTRACT: In medical training, allowing learners to take pauses during tasks is known to enhance performance. Cognitive load theory assumes that insertion of pauses positively affects cognitive load, thereby enhancing performance. However, empirical studies on how allowing and taking pauses affects cognitive load and performance in dynamic task environments are scarce. We investigated the pause effect, using a computerised simulation game in emergency medicine. Medical students (N = 70) were randomly assigned to one of two conditions: simulation with (n = 40) and without (n = 30) the option to take pauses. All participants played the same two scenarios, during which game logs and eye-tracking data were recorded. Overall, both cognitive load and performance were higher in the condition with pauses than in the one without. The act of pausing, however, temporarily lowered cognitive load, especially during intense moments. Two different manifestations of the pause effect were identified: (1) by stimulating additional cognitive and meta-cognitive processes, pauses increased overall cognitive load; and (2) through relaxation, the act of pausing temporarily decreased heightened cognitive load. Consequently, our results suggest that in order to enhance students' performance and learning it is important that we encourage them to utilise the different effects of pausing.

In actuality, there are a number of ways to perform a 'constructive pause' including:

O - Thought Transfer or Thought Pause

O - Level 1 Meditation - The Body Scan

O - Breathing For A Relaxation Pause

**In this book, I am talking about the HACK I have found to be the most effective technique; The 'Thought Transfer' or 'Thought Pause' (and no, I am not talking about ESP or anything like that)**

I'll start by explaining how you do one:

1. Prepare by scheduling a 5 to 10 minute break in your morning, and one again in your afternoon (ideally at least 4 hours apart)

2. Get a pen and paper ready for each session

3. At the scheduled time, find a quiet place to sit where you will not be disturbed.

4. Turn off or silence all devices

5. Start a 3 minute timer

6. Write down ALL thoughts which come to mind, no matter how trivial

7. Stop when the timer ends

8. Keep the list safe

9. Return to your day's activities

In the afternoon, when your scheduled 2nd session is due, repeat the steps as before:

1. Get a pen and paper ready for each session

2. At the scheduled time, find a quiet place to sit where you will not be disturbed.

3. Turn off or silence all devices

4. Start a 3 minute timer

5. Write down ALL thoughts which come to mind, no matter how trivial

6. Stop when the timer ends

This time, before you return to your day's activities, compare the items on the two lists, this one and the one from the morning session.

You might notice that many of the initial items on the first list are not on the latest one. Most people do, but if you don't, not to worry as it can take a good few sessions for some, before the 'magic' starts happening!

This is a little known but very effective exercise, which uses the psychological concept of letting your brain release certain thoughts when they are tangibly written or recorded somewhere.

Now you might be thinking this is just another 'to-do' list, and the use of 'notes' or 'to-do' lists is well known to help people not to forget important things, but they are generally random, unstructured and unfocused.

The magic 'Secret' I discovered, is that rather than using notes to avoid forgetting things, by actually formalising the exercise by following the above steps every time, your brain established a 'pattern' (and brains work on neural patterns) which allows it to let go of the things written down, as it accepts that there is then an 'external map' of those thoughts.

In actuality, there are a number of ways to perform a 'constructive pause' including:

O - Thought Transfer or Thought Pause

O - Level 1 Meditation - The Body Scan

O - Breathing For A Relaxation Pause

**In this book, I am talking about the HACK I have found to be the most effective technique; The 'Thought Transfer' or 'Thought Pause' (and no, I am not talking about ESP or anything like that)**

I'll start by explaining how you do one:

1.  Prepare by scheduling a 5 to 10 minute break in your morning, and one again in your afternoon (ideally at least 4 hours apart)

2.  Get a pen and paper ready for each session

3.  At the scheduled time, find a quiet place to sit where you will not be disturbed.

4.  Turn off or silence all devices

5.  Start a 3 minute timer

6.  Write down ALL thoughts which come to mind, no matter how trivial

7.  Stop when the timer ends

8.  Keep the list safe

9.  Return to your day's activities

In the afternoon, when your scheduled 2nd session is due, repeat the steps as before:

1. Get a pen and paper ready for each session

2. At the scheduled time, find a quiet place to sit where you will not be disturbed.

3. Turn off or silence all devices

4. Start a 3 minute timer

5. Write down ALL thoughts which come to mind, no matter how trivial

6. Stop when the timer ends

This time, before you return to your day's activities, compare the items on the two lists, this one and the one from the morning session.

You might notice that many of the initial items on the first list are not on the latest one. Most people do, but if you don't, not to worry as it can take a good few sessions for some, before the 'magic' starts happening!

This is a little known but very effective exercise, which uses the psychological concept of letting your brain release certain thoughts when they are tangibly written or recorded somewhere.

Now you might be thinking this is just another 'to-do' list, and the use of 'notes' or 'to-do' lists is well known to help people not to forget important things, but they are generally random, unstructured and unfocused.

The magic 'Secret' I discovered, is that rather than using notes to avoid forgetting things, by actually formalising the exercise by following the above steps every time, your brain established a 'pattern' (and brains work on neural patterns) which allows it to let go of the things written down, as it accepts that there is then an 'external map' of those thoughts.

In essence we are actually making the brain forget them, so the reverse of the 'to-do' list! Why are we doing this?

Well, the thoughts first written down in almost every list, are almost always the smaller less important ones. The ones taking up valuable resources and interfering with the bigger issues which need all your brain power (which is severely limited, by the way, and you can learn more about that in my upcoming latest book "Burnout Hacking Secrets" or in my Cognitive Masterclass Training) in order to get resolved.

By moving the little thoughts out of the way, you can identify and then deal with the big ones, and THEY are the ones that are causing the stress and sleepless nights!

One person on one of my courses, found that by doing this hack regularly, their productivity had gone through the roof, as they were hitting all the top issues quickly and effectively, and using the process to manage all the little things 'off-brain', as I call it.

Try it for yourself, and see your own efficiency rise, regardless of whether it is at work or at home/play!

The more often you carry out this exercise, (within reason!) the more you can identify and then apply focus to those issues which are the most important.

The story of how I ultimately discovered this hack is not a glamorous one, but one of HUNDREDS of hours of learning and research.

After forming the idea from the research I referenced above, I also discovered a study by Deshmukh, V. D. (2014), looking at the effects of rumination on the cognitive functioning, and how it reacted to meditation and creative activities, which identified that human attention functions in two modes: vector mode (predominantly cognitive) and matrix mode (predominantly presence or existential awareness).

The process of Cognitive Pause-and-Unload (CPU) involves pausing and disengaging this cognitive mode (vector-attention) and unloading the cognitive contents from the working memory.

At this point, you remain intrinsically aware and receptive to the reality in the present (matrix mode ground-state of attentiveness).

Now, a creative process typically has four phases:

1. Preparation, 2. Incubation, 3. Illumination, and 4. Verification.

The CPU process deepens and enhances the incubation period, which then reshuffles and refreshes the contents of working memory. This may result in a new idea, a novel design, or an innovative solution, in much the way we tend to come up with solutions once we stop thinking so much about the issue, often in the shower for example.

Whilst the study goes on to consider meditation as an attention-emotion training regime leading to mental calm, clarity and creativity, I began looking at this from the opposite direction, namely deliberately applying pauses to allow that 'buffer' time to rest the cognitive (vector-attention) energy hungry part of our brain, so as to allow us to 'come back to the issue' later with a 'fresh mind', and typically discover those novel creative solutions we need.

In a number of other studies, focus was being placed on the purpose of observed pausing in translation activities, and why the brain was doing this, and again, I felt I should approach this from a different perspective, as it seemed to me their brains were 'telling' them something about how it needed to insert rests in order to operate effectively.

I had 'reversed' the focus on to deliberate activation of a 'pause' rather than observing when they happened, to improve cognitive performance across a longer period of time, like a working day, and found performance was universally improved, albeit across a wide scale of results, but still all positive.

"And what has this to do with Peak Performance?" I hear you ask...

Well, the most research into this comes from sports science, and the drive to deliver peak physical and mental performance when needed, particularly during high level events.

Being able to deliver that all important aggression, or calm the mind and body in order to not seize up during a longer period of optimum performance, is critical for top level sports people, and they manage this through techniques to effectively control their emotional and physical arousal (Arousal Control)

Think about the following images. They show the two extremes of Arousal Control. The first, a calming method to reduce the arousal and get themselves under complete control:

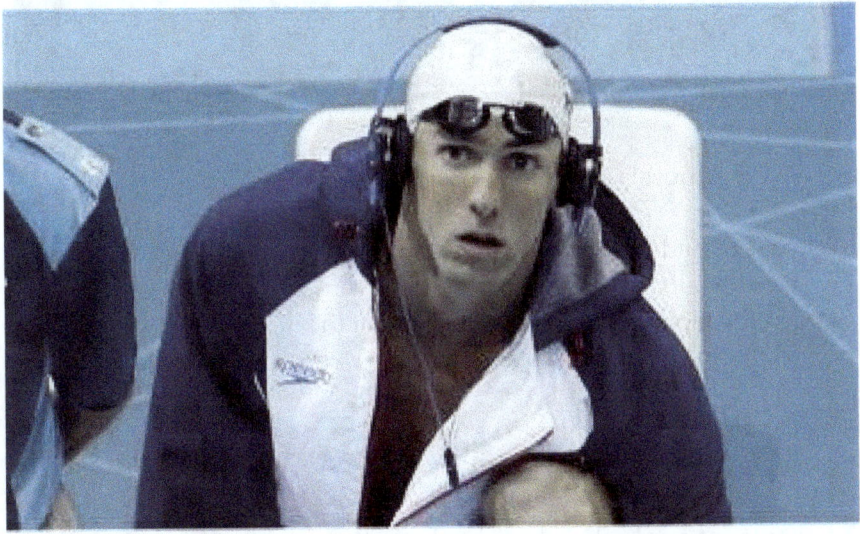

The second a method of increasing arousal in preparation for an explosive effort:

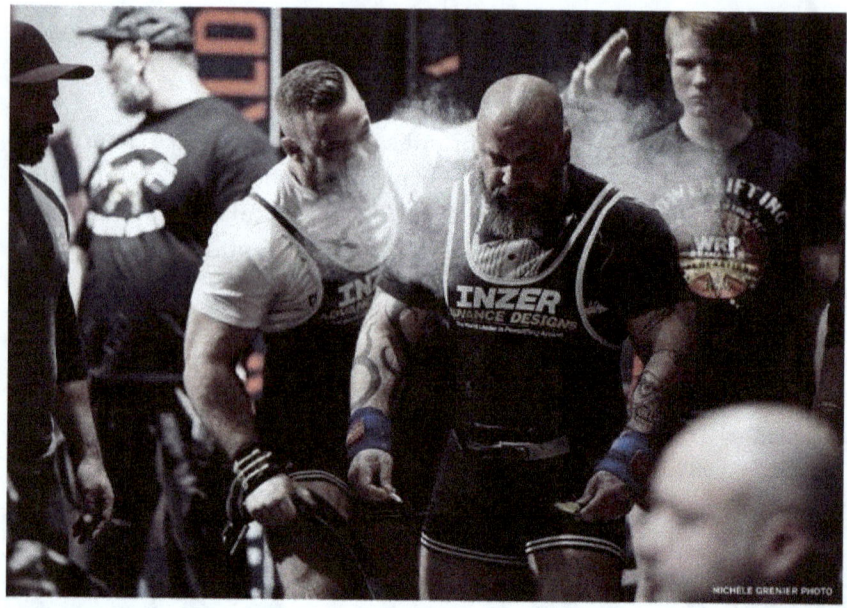

So, why is Arousal Control important to us generally?

We have all had experience of situations when we have not been in the best emotional state for an impending event or activity. Lethargy first thing in the morning or towards the end of the day, and over excitement or anxiety when heading to an important event or meeting.

This can find us struggling to be 'present' or to maintain a clear thought process under pressure.

To operate at our best, we need to be in the 'sweet spot' or 'Goldilocks Zone' of the Arousal Control Inverted U Graph, making sure we are neither under nor over aroused.

## There is a 'Sweet Spot' for emotional arousal...

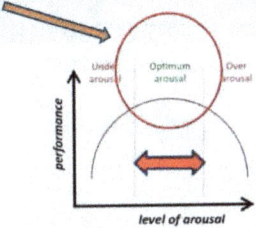

*This is the range within which we are able to focus and have high levels of energy, but are not anxious or panicky, caused by our System 1 (reactive and impulsive) taking control and preventing optimally balanced processing of crystallised and fluid intelligence.*

**To REDUCE our arousal, one of the best 'hacks' is the '4-7-8 Breathing Technique'!**

There have been many variations of this timing, but repeated research has found the optimum combination is to execute this technique as follows:

1 - Breath in through your nose, filling your lungs in 4 seconds

2 - Hold that breath for 7 seconds

3 - Breath out through your mouth for 8 seconds

4 - Repeat a number of times!

What this is doing physiologically to our body, is covered in more detail in my Masterclass, but it is essentially a calming technique, optimised for arousal control.

For INCREASING our arousal, such as to 'kick-start' the day, or get us 'fired-up' for something like an important meeting, there are other techniques and approaches like exercise, coffee or caffeine drinks, and rapid breath exercises.

Now in order to be operating at our best, it is not just our arousal levels that need to be managed, but also any negative thinking we may have, and in my training course, I cover techniques for managing negative self-talk.

## There is a 'Sweet Spot' for emotional arousal...

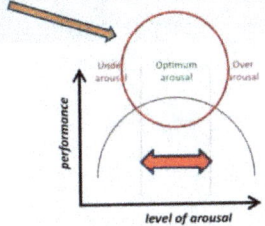

*This is the range within which we are able to focus and have high levels of energy, but are not anxious or panicky, caused by our System 1 (reactive and impulsive) taking control and preventing optimally balanced processing of crystallised and fluid intelligence.*

**To REDUCE our arousal, one of the best 'hacks' is the '4-7-8 Breathing Technique'!**

There have been many variations of this timing, but repeated research has found the optimum combination is to execute this technique as follows:

1 - Breath in through your nose, filling your lungs in 4 seconds

2 - Hold that breath for 7 seconds

3 - Breath out through your mouth for 8 seconds

4 - Repeat a number of times!

What this is doing physiologically to our body, is covered in more detail in my Masterclass, but it is essentially a calming technique, optimised for arousal control.

For INCREASING our arousal, such as to 'kick-start' the day, or get us 'fired-up' for something like an important meeting, there are other techniques and approaches like exercise, coffee or caffeine drinks, and rapid breath exercises.

Now in order to be operating at our best, it is not just our arousal levels that need to be managed, but also any negative thinking we may have, and in my training course, I cover techniques for managing negative self-talk.

## Neuroscience In Leadership...

Dr David Rock once said:

*"Start every meeting with complete clarity on what the objective is. Work out what your goal is, what you're going toward. Then work out the best plan to get there, and be sure to foster a sense of clarity and alignment with everyone involved. Whether you're in a meeting or having a conversation, be clear on the purpose and the plan. Throughout this process, continue to notice the quality of your thinking along the way--be meta-cognitive."*

He was discussing the need to have as much certainty in your OWN thinking processes as much as being cognisant of the information which is flowing around you.

Part of this self-knowledge relates to understanding your own cognitive landscape.

Remember the concept of 'Brain-Lateralisation' I covered in 'The Brain & Intelligence'? This was about the Left and Right Hemispheres, which deal with logical and creative thinking.

To expand a bit more, your RIGHT side is:

* Biased towards a physical, emotional self.

* Superior at synthesising information at a preconscious level to provide

an overall sense or picture of something.

* Responds to emotionally laden information and intense pre-verbal emotional processes, faster to incoming stimuli than the left.

* The Right Amygdala is biased towards negative emotions.

* Heightened activation of right sided structures is caused by stress and anxiety.

Your LEFT side, comparatively, is:

* Biased towards the conscious self.

* Specialising in cognitive tasks such as problem solving, conscious coping and language.

* Superior at managing detailed tasks.

* Responds to cognitive information more slowly, indicating that emotion (right hemisphere) precedes thinking.

* The Left Amygdala is biased towards positive emotions

Did you know you have a dominant side? Are you left or right hemisphere dominant? How can you find out?

A quick way is to consider the following:

- Which ear would you use to listen at a door with?

- Which eye is your stronger?

- Which hand is dominant?

- Which foot would you use to kick a ball?

If you answers include more Right's than Left's then you are **Left**

**Brained,** and conversely more Left's than Right's means you are **Right Brained.** In my Cognitive Masterclass I have a cool game which works out your eye dominance!

There are a whole bunch of chemical processes going on during periods of stress.

Cortisol release is triggered, which is natural, but prolonged periods of **overproduction** of cortisol has a harmful effect, including cognitive changes such as memory degradation and depression, as well as a reduction in the size of the Hippocampus, caused by this level of cortisol destroying neurons in greater numbers than the natural process. This is important because the Hippocampus is the area in your brain central to processing memory

Cortisol also causes over-activity in the pre-frontal cortex, resulting in reactions such as fearfulness, irritability and social withdrawal, and also inhibition of the regulating functions of the pre-frontal cortex, leading to difficulties in managing behaviours, reactions, emotions and thinking processes.

Effects of this neuroscience on our behaviours can be seen in a number of cognitive structures and experiences:

1. Fear

*Fear is an Emotional Reaction, processed by our limbic brain, specifically the Amygdala. The limbic brain and Amygdala is oriented towards perceiving threats and negative events, and is a self-preservation system, created during our early development as a species, so it is extremely quick at responding. The problem is that this is a reactive and impulsive system, subject to acting without thinking, operating too fast for our pre-frontal cortex to consider the reality or extent of any threat, meaning the threat assessment is quite often over-estimated by today's standards.*

2. Fragmentation

*Memory is actually the storage of patterns of activity, created and strengthened* when groups of neurons fire together. These patterns are fragmented, by being stored and distributed across different parts of the brain, in different memory systems. It is because of this fragmentation, that memories have to be reconstructed every time they are retrieved, causing certain peripheral details to change in a 'memory' each time it is recalled.

3. Memory Types

*We actually have 2 types of memory, namely 'explicit' and 'implicit, with the implicit memory stored in our limbic brain as 'unconscious memory'. When we are in a similar physical or emotional situation as an original one where a memory was first established, we use something called 'state-dependent retrieval', which is where we recall that previous experience, enabling us to react quickly rather than re-learn it every time, which is obviously a much slower process with longer reaction times. The problem with this is that it can encourage impulsive and reactive behaviours, rather than considered responses which take into account the present information, if we don't apply our Impulse Control (see earlier chapter) and allow the pre-frontal cortex to be engaged.*

When we look at the application of knowledge gained from social neuroscientific research on behaviours, there appears to be two clear themes emerging. Firstly, that much of our motivation driving social behaviour is governed by an overarching organising principle of minimising threat and maximising reward. Secondly, that several domains of social experience draw upon the **same brain networks** to maximise reward and minimise threat, as the brain networks used for primary survival needs. What this means is that social needs are treated in much the same way in the brain as the need for food and water.

Within Leadership, it is important to recognise and understand the application of this knowledge, and tailor our behaviours accordingly.

For example, although a job is often regarded as a purely economic transaction, in which people exchange their efforts for financial compensation, the brain experiences the workplace first and foremost as a **social system**. Leaders who understand this dynamic can more effectively engage their employees' best talents, support collaborative teams, and create an environment that fosters productive change. **In**

**fact, the HACK here is the ability to intentionally address the social brain in the service of optimal performance, which will be a distinguishing leadership capability more and more coveted in senior leadership roles, as our understanding of management and relationship dynamics develops further.**

The impact of this neural dynamic is very often visible in organisations, once you know what to look for, such as a so-called 'Jekyll & Hyde Effect'. For example, when (Hyde) leaders trigger a threat response (I cover 'Threat' and 'Reward' responses in more detail in my Cognitive Masterclass), employees' brains become much less efficient. However, when (Jekyll) leaders make people feel good about themselves, clearly communicate their expectations, give employees latitude to make decisions, support people's efforts to build good relationships, and treat the whole organisation fairly, it prompts a reward response. This 'Jekyll' behaviour finds others in the organisation becoming more effective, more open to ideas and more creative. They begin to notice the kind of information that they miss when fear or resentment, under a 'Hyde' leader, makes it difficult to focus their attention. What is important from a Burnout (mental health) perspective, is that with a 'Jekyll' leader, workers are less susceptible to workplace stress related burnout, because they generally experience lower stress levels through the product of feeling more intrinsically rewarded.

For leaders, every action you take and every decision you make either supports or undermines your workforce's perceived levels of status, certainty, autonomy, relatedness and fairness in your enterprise. In fact, this is why leading is considered so difficult. It is critical to know the drivers that can cause a threat response, as this enables you, as a leader, to knowingly deliver interactions to minimise threats.

A problem exists, however, in the form of the imbalance between threat & reward responses. In a study by Kyle Benson in 2017, he established what he called 'The Magic Relationship Ratio', which is the balance needed of positive to negative interactions in good effective relationships during times of conflict, to be 5:1, meaning our brains apply 5 times as much impact to threat responses as reward responses. In simplistic terms, we need 5 rewards to counter 1 threat.

It is worth understanding that our typical reaction to the strong negative emotions generated by a threat response is to suppress them, particularly in the workplace, however this response has many undesirable consequences, from reducing our own memory function to raising the blood pressure of people around us, so the cost of a threat response doesn't impact solely by the person experiencing it, but anyone who interacts with them or depends on their effectiveness. In essence it's a shared social experience, and this highlights the importance of group dynamics, perhaps most significantly, the extent to which it's safe (or unsafe) in a given group to express negative or difficult emotions. Something very much in the spotlight of behavioural possibilities in our working environments, today.

To makes things all the more challenging, we have approximately 1/3 of a second after the perception of a potential threat, before a neurological threat response is triggered. That is the time we have to apply our impulse control HACK from before, so not a lot! This means on an individual basis, and this is the supporting HACK here (Yes. You get 2 for 1 in this section!), it's essential to develop and improve our ability to recognise the conditions that might trigger a threat response, and proactively reappraise the situation, and at the group or interpersonal level, it's important to be aware of the speed and ease with which a threat response can be triggered in someone else, to understand how such a response is likely to undermine effective communication, and to take steps that support the other person's reappraisal of the situation without creating defensiveness. **This is Emotional Intelligence (Your EQ).**

## *Communicating With EQ (your emotional intelligence) ...*

Having now learnt a little about neuroscience and its affects on our brains and behaviours, as well as how leaders should be looking to apply this in how they serve their staff, and maximise their productivity, we can focus this down a bit onto how to use it in our communication with others.

Dr David Rock explored the field of neuroscience and its implications for management, coaching, and organisational life, and established a hugely effective framework for understanding the five primary social dimensions within which our brains respond to perceived threats and rewards, which has now been well established, worldwide.

He called it the SCARF model and it summarises the two themes we identified in the last chapter, namely that we prioritise reducing threats and increasing rewards, and that the parts of the brain which deal with these responses compete for the same neural maps in its various parts, within a framework that captures the common factors that can activate a reward or threat response in social situations.

This model has been tested and proven by many, myself included, in any situation where people collaborate in groups, including all types of workplaces, educational environments, family settings and general social events.

This increases the value of learning and understanding the model, to be valid in any aspect of your life, and not just consign it to another business tool which appears to be only relevant to managers.

**The SCARF model, which is the HACK here, involves five domains of human social experience:**

*S* **- Status (relative importance to others)**

*C* **- Certainty (being able to predict the future)**

*A* **- Autonomy (a sense of control over events)**

*R* **- Relatedness (a sense of safety with others)**

*F* **- Fairness (perception of fair exchange between people)**

These five domains activate either the "primary reward" or "primary threat" circuitry (and associated networks) of the brain. For example, a perceived threat to one's status activates similar brain networks to a threat to one's life. In the same way, a perceived increase in fairness activates the same reward circuitry as receiving a monetary reward.

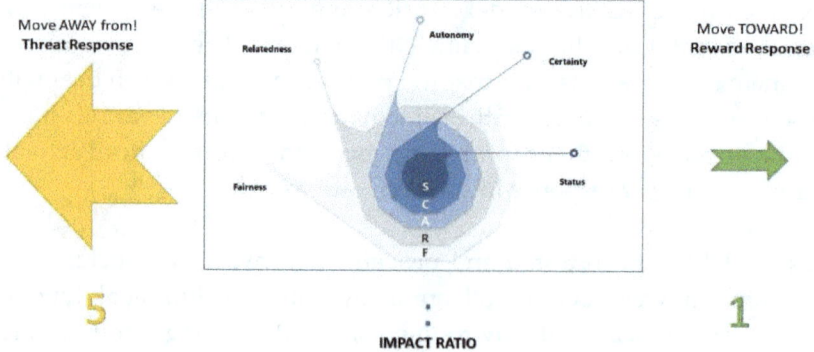

These are all connected to our response mechanisms, and as you can see from the diagram, the unconscious drive to move away from 'threats' is greater than our move towards rewards, and is part of our 'self-preservation' system, and it is here you can see Kyle Benson's 'Magic Relationship Ratio' of 5:1 *(5 Rewards needed to balance 1 Threat)*, in action.

When you consider that **Status** is about perceived relative importance, position and seniority, you can see that it is important that extreme care be taken to conduct reviews and provide feedback in ways designed to boost, rather than threaten, the recipient's status, but also that attention must be paid to the small, commonplace ways in which interpersonal status is heightened and diminished. Of course this doesn't have to be just in the workplace, but equally important in personal relationships and communication.

Now, the brain is in a constant quest to conserve energy, which derives from the limited capacity of the pre-frontal cortex, the centre of our cognitive executive functioning. We naturally resist mental effort around decision-making and impulse control, because we're preserving resources in case we need them more urgently in the next moment, and this same dynamic contributes to our resistance to uncertainty. When we lack **certainty** and can't predict what will happen next, the brain has to apply significantly more resources to process moment-to-moment experiences, so when **perceived** uncertainty gets out of hand, people tend to panic and make bad decisions.

When we think about how much **autonomy** we consider we have, this perception of our ability to exert control over our environment has a substantial effect on our response to stress factors in our life. When we feel more autonomous and able to control a situation, we're much more resistant to stress. There is a clear interplay across many of these, for example when we believe we have more autonomy and control, we feel more certainty in the moment and the immediate future. It should be noted that meaningful perceptions of autonomy can be generated by small gestures, however subtle, and this perception of autonomy can be used to help people manage stress better.

When we think of **Relatedness,** it is often described as "the ability to feel trust and empathy about others" and this is shaped by whether they are perceived to be part of the same social group. When a new person enters our life, if they are perceived as different, the information travels along neural pathways that are associated with uncomfortable feelings (different from those triggered by people who are perceived as similar to oneself.) Once people begin to make a stronger social connection, their brains begin to secrete a hormone called oxytocin in one another's presence, and from a neuroscientific perspective, this process allows our brains to classify the other person as "friend" rather than "foe," and contributes to establishing feelings of trust and empathy. So in an interpersonal setting it's important to interact in ways that will surface points of similarity, strengthen social connections and increase a sense of relatedness.

The final element is fairness, and neuroscience tells us that if there is a perception that an event has been unfair, this generates a strong response in the brain, stirring hostility and undermining trust. It has been found that perceived unfair exchanges generate a strong threat response which can sometimes include activation of the insular, a part of the brain involved in intense emotions such as disgust. Just like status, perceptions of fairness are relative, and what YOU think of as being unfair, the other(s) in the situation may not, which leads to conflict. As a rule, it is better to stop trying to convince the other side of your 'rightness' and simply accept your relative perceptions, if you want to make any progress toward resolving your differences.

In my Masterclass, I go into more detail around the SCARF elements, but for now, let's look at how these lessons can be applied to the way we communicate - Applying The HACK!

Consider the following workplace scenario:

A number of minor collisions have occurred in the management car-park, and there has been an announcement made by the Health & Safety Director which reads as follows:

*As you may be aware, a number of incidents have happened in the car-park due to some of you not following the clearly signed directional signage. I cannot understand how it is that as managers you seem incapable of following simple* instructions.

As a member of the Executive team, this makes me have to consider your suitability as manager material, as you are expected to be a role model.

With immediate effect, access to the car park will be restricted to one entry to enforce the directional instructions.

I am disappointed that I have to explain this to people of your seniority.

Any further contraventions seen on CCTV footage will result in immediate loss of parking privileges.

I have, of course, structured this message to easily apply the SCARF model, and would suggest before reading on, that you see how you would break the message down yourself.

Here is how it breaks down under the SCARF categories:

```
STATUS: As you may be aware, a number of
incidents have happened in the car-park due to
some of you not following the clearly signed
directional signage. I cannot understand how it
is that as managers you seem incapable of
following simple instructions.

CERTAINTY: As a member of the Executive team,
this makes me have to consider your suitability
as manager material, as you are expected to be a
role model.

AUTONOMY: With immediate effect, access to the
car park will be restricted to one entry to
enforce the directional instructions.

RELATEDNESS: I am disappointed that I have to
explain this to people of your seniority.

FAIRNESS: Any further contraventions seen on cctv
footage will result in immediate loss of parking
```

*privileges.*

If you were one of the managers in this scenario and received this message, how would you feel? Not great I suspect!

If we take the message and apply the core elements of Dr Rock's framework, we could change this to read more like the following:

*As you may be aware, a number of minor incidents have happened recently in the car-park, and you have all been selected as championing a new 'driving safely' initiative, because we believe in your professionalism and understanding of safety in all areas of the workplace.*

*We are proud to have strong role models in our management, and value your influence.*

*We would like to hear any suggestions you may have individually or as a collective, on how to improve safety in this parking area.*

*If you need anything to help us reach our mutual goal of higher safety, please feel free to contact the Executive Team.*

*We would like to establish an ongoing dialogue and feedback between us, to ensure every voice is heard.*

The message is inherently still unchanged, in that a reduction in accidents and increase in safety is needed, but consider how you would feel if you received THIS message instead of the original?

Does it support or undermine your status? Is there any question over certainty of your job security or position? Do you feel your personal control (autonomy) over the activity has been eroded or enhanced? Are you feeling part of the company and included in the 'social group' of the workforce? Does the approach seem fair or unfair?

There are other models, which I cover in my Masterclass, which are simpler in construct, which are easier to implement in different types of working environment where using SCARF might be a bit too complex and onerous to apply consistently, like my RACE model approach **(HACK #2)** shown in the diagram below.

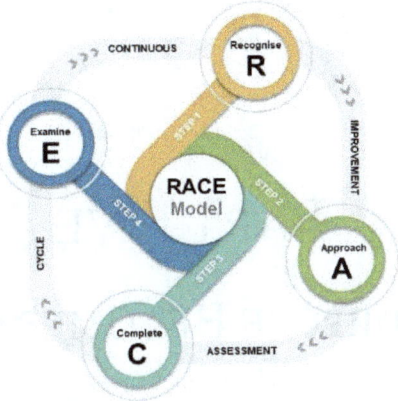

Using these HACKS not only helps your own levels of stress and anxiety, in this case as a manager of people, but it also helps those with whom you interact as a bonus!

# Part Five

## My Purpose Becomes Clear

## *Sharing The Knowledge...*

Having been through the 'Trauma' and despite losing so much, surviving almost intact, I believed my purpose was to take the knowledge I had gained from the years of research and testing, and go round and coach and impart this knowledge to companies and organisations, in the hope that they would implement some form of ongoing training as part of their induction process for all new employees, and retro-train all existing staff.

What I found was that, whilst I was hugely busy doing these workshops and training up to 10 at a time to understand what I had learned would help prevent the rate of burnout within their businesses, I was just scratching the surface and needed to seriously increase the coverage.

It was a serendipitous moment when one of the 'students' from a workshop asked if they could train to be able to deliver this themselves. It was literally within a few days of my 'realisation' moment.

I considered it a sign, and began creating my coaching course for Burnout Prevention Educators, which would not just provide them with all the knowledge they needed, but also with the skills to create their own materials and, more importantly, deliver this in various environments and using various medium.

Taking the original workshop materials, I created an extended train-the-trainer course and a certification exam, allowing the attendees to choose to certify if they wanted to join my growing network of 'educators'.

At this point, I also took the in-person workshop materials, and restructured them into on-line course sessions (over 8 hours worth), and offered a further coaching enhancement to my certified students, to develop this and deliver it themselves.

It quickly became obvious that, whilst the group was growing and the message was organically spreading through more and more trained coaches, I needed to do more.

I had to do 2 things:

Firstly, teach my coaches to train other coaches, and secondly, coach those who wanted it (which turned out to be many) how to set up their own business to deliver this training, both to end users and to 'new trainers'

## *Establishing The Business...*

I had a great growing group of coaches and coach trainers, who were all fantastic at delivering the knowledge and educating anybody who came across their path, but there was a lack of a foundational banner under which we all could march.

At this point, BURNOUT-HACKER.COM was born!

Prior to this I had been operating under my N Cubed Group Company, using the 'My Better Life Coaching' brand under its umbrella, but that was an identity which had a different specific purpose, and so I needed to create a strong banner under which we all marched.

I spent a long while considering what we were actually doing, that was both past and future proofed, and realised after some months of many discussions with, frankly anyone who would listen, that I was still 100% focused and passionate about hacking the path to burnout, so that nobody need experience the horrendous traumas I had, and then the name was just plainly obvious.

**I AM A BURNOUT HACKER!**

My training will help anyone avoid the impacts of burnout on themselves and their loved ones! Simple as that!

Now I just needed to accelerate the distribution of this ability and effectiveness of the time I spent training and coaching others to do this.

## *Creating The Ultimate Retreat...*

Being passionate about anything will typically drive you to find the quickest and most efficient way of achieving your goals, and so I set to work out how I could condense ALL the training, coaching and education into as short a period as possible, but lose none of its impact or quality.

The answer was, in the end, easy.

An intense, full on, 'soup to nuts' retreat!

I hold up to 4 of these a year, in various places around the world, and they tend to sell out within about an hour these days.

Now, these are not for everyone.

For one thing, they are on the face of it expensive, although not when you understand the value of what you get.

Second, they are VERY intense, held usually over 5 days, during which I cram in ALL the education, coaching, train-the-trainer coaching, business set up AND full coaching on direct marketing! You can literally come away with everything you need for kicking off your first sessions, through your own business! (IF you have kept up and put the effort in). For some it may take a few weeks extra to complete all the tasks, before they reach the same point, but that is typically just because other stuff gets in the way!

If you want to get direct coaching from me, this is now the only way to achieve it at this level. It is only for my Platinum Club Members.

I have had over 140 go through this so far (at time of writing) and not a single one has ever said they didn't get fantastic value from the cost of the retreat!

These people are all now personal friends, and are jointly involved in the constant reshaping and extending of the knowledge shared and delivered through Burnout Prevention Education globally.

**They are all BURNOUT HACKERS!**

Come join us. I'd love to see you there!

# PART SIX

## WHAT NOW?

## *My Hopes For You...*

I hope this book serves you in two ways:

Firstly, you understand the potentially massive impact a real burnout can have, not only on the individual, but in many ways more importantly, on their family and loved ones.

Secondly, that you embrace the secret 'Hacks' I have described, and protect yourself and your loved ones from similar experiences as mine.

I personally get huge satisfaction and pride in teaching my Masterclasses, because I know I have given every participant the tools and techniques to make sure they protect and even strengthen their cognitive resilience and performance, often leading to lifestyle improvements through promotions and better life/work balance.

I would love for you to come and join us in spreading this knowledge, either in your own workplace, or by setting up your OWN business to do so, which I also can help with if you choose to do so.

I look forward to seeing you in one of my sessions, or even at one of my exclusive RETREATS!

Find out more at: *burnout-hacker.com* or by emailing me at *laurence@burnout-hacker.com*.

# PART SEVEN

## HACKS LIST

## *Summary Of The Hacks In This Book...*

#1 - Cognitive Hack for extending Fluid Intelligence: Continued 'exercising' of what Hercule Poirot called the 'little grey cells', across the appropriate cognitive skills, can delay the onset of decline and reduce the gradient and ultimate intersection point of the crystallised and fluid intelligence gradients. (See section: The Brain & Intelligence)

#2 - One of the best 'hacks' for exercising and improving our impulse control, is the Stroop Test (explained in detail in my Cognitive Masterclass), and one many people are probably already familiar with, where words describing colours (red, blue, green, etc.) are flashed either on cards or on screen, but with the font also displayed in a colour, which might be different to the colour the word is describing, for example the word RED might be shown but displayed in BLUE ink/screen colour. (See section: Impulse Control)

#3 - How can you 'hack' your brain and create an environment to assist in improving your ability to focus your attention? Exercises! Focus exercises! There are methods which make you focus and ignore external distractions, such as memory 'journey' exercises, which force you to spend longer focusing on remembering a set of steps, which in turn improves both your recall from working memory and your ability to 'zone out' local distractions. (See section: Attention)

#4 - The HACK I have found to be the most effective technique for Constructive Pausing; The 'Thought Transfer' or 'Thought Pause'. (See section: Pauses, Peak Performance & Arousal Control)

#5 - To REDUCE our arousal, one of the best 'hacks' is the '4-7-8 Breathing Technique'! (See section: Pauses, Peak Performance & Arousal Control)

#6 - The HACK for applying Neuroscience to Leadership Behaviours is the ability to intentionally address the social brain in the service of optimal performance, which will be a distinguishing leadership capability more and more coveted in senior leadership roles, as our understanding of management and relationship dynamics develops further. The supporting HACK here (Yes. You get 2 for 1 in this section!), it's essential to develop and improve our ability to recognise the conditions that might trigger a threat response, and proactively reappraise the situation, and at the group or interpersonal level, it's important to be aware of the speed and ease with which a threat response can be triggered in someone else, to understand how such a response is likely to undermine effective communication, and to take steps that support the other person's reappraisal of the situation without creating defensiveness. (See section: Neuroscience in Leadership)

#7 - For communication using EQ, the HACK here is The SCARF model, which involves the five domains of human social experience; STATUS, CERTAINTY, AUTONOMY, RELATEDNESS and FAIRNESS. (See section: Communicating with EQ)

# Part Eight
## Bonus Secrets

## *Stress & Anxiety...*

Considering almost all burnouts, especially workplace stress triggered ones, are caused by Stress and Anxiety, there are a number of well known methods for reducing both of these, BUT it is actually less about the approach but more about the implementation, where the real power lays. **The 'Secrets' or HACKS lay in the <u>WAY you carry out the elements</u>, not the elements themselves, which are fairly widely accepted already, as methods of reducing your levels of stress and anxiety.**

**Buster #1 - Exercise**

"Any type of exercise can increase your fitness and decrease your stress. However, it's important to choose an activity that you enjoy rather than dread."

It is well known that exercise can improve your physical health, trim your body, improve your sex life, and even add years to your life. Any or all of these benefits are offered as the reasons most people give for starting to exercise, but it is rarely what motivates most people to stay active.

It has been found that those who exercise regularly tend to do so because of a great sense of well-being felt from doing so. They feel more energetic throughout the day, sleep better at night, have sharper memories, and feel more relaxed and positive about themselves and their lives. On top of this, it can also be powerful medicine for many common mental health challenges.

There are noticeable symptoms felt within yourself when you are under stress, specifically including tension in the muscles in your face, neck, and shoulders, which often leaves you with back or neck pain, or painful headaches. Other typical stress symptoms include: a pounding pulse, muscle cramps, insomnia, heartburn, stomach ache, diarrhoea, or frequently needing to 'wee'.

As well as releasing 'pleasure' chemicals called 'endorphins' in the brain, physical activity helps to relax the muscles and relieve tension in the body. Since the body and mind are so closely linked, when your body feels better so, too, will your mind.

Always check with your GP before starting, but there are a whole range of options available out there.

You don't need to be a marathon runner or elite athlete to experience stress relief from exercise. Almost any kind of exercise can be helpful.

For example, consider trying moderate aerobic exercises such as:

> cycling

> brisk walking or jogging

> swimming or doing water aerobics

> playing a racket sport

> dancing

> rowing

When it comes to muscle-strengthening exercises, consider trying weight lifting or activities with resistance bands.

Even something as simple as gardening or choosing to take the stairs rather than the elevator can give you an emotional lift.

**The HACK: Any type of exercise can increase your fitness and decrease your stress, but choose an activity that you enjoy rather than dread.**

**Doing something you don't enjoy won't help relieve your stress. Try a variety of activities until you find some you enjoy.**

**When you're having fun, you'll be more likely to stick with your workout routine.**

**Buster #2 - Breathing**

"When a person is under stress, their breathing pattern changes usually to small, shallow breaths, and this shallow over-breathing, or hyperventilation, can prolong feelings of anxiety by making the physical symptoms of stress worse."

We have all been there at some point in our lives, and many more than once; the sudden increase in heart rate, the increase in body temperature, the feeling of lightheadedness.

The causes can be numerous, but all share a common theme: we are facing something unknown or something we fear in some way, or have exhausted our cognitive capacity and we are resorting to reactive protective pre-conditioning.

It can be an upcoming presentation at work, or a strange noise in the night, or an oncoming person or group of people who look intimidating, all of which trigger our 'Freeze - Flight - Fight' response. This age old survival mechanism is not required much these days in the way it was for our distant ancestors, but even though our environment is very different to way back then, the response can still be valid, especially if feeling threatened.

Often, though, this is an overreaction in today's environments, and we need to have a way of 'turning off' the automatic (limbic) response by recognising the fear is not as we believe it to be.

**The HACK: Controlling your breathing can help to improve some of these symptoms should you feel an anxiety or panic attack coming on:**

- **Apply the 4-7-8 Breathing technique. When you feel your breath quickening, focus your attention on inhaling through your nose for 4 seconds, holding this full breath for 7 seconds, and then slowly exhale through your mouth for 8 seconds. Repeat until your breathing slows. This is extremely effective for those pre-presentation or interview anxiety nerves.**

A couple more techniques you can try for yourselves should you find the symptoms of anxiety building, include:

- Recognise and accept what you're experiencing. If you've already experienced an anxiety or panic attack, you know that it can be incredibly frightening. Remind yourself that the symptoms will pass and you'll be alright. Also, that the level of perceived threat is not usually accurate and that this response is not required, as the situation is rarely as threatening as you believe. Repeating this in a type of mantra can help to reduce your stress response.

- Practice mindfulness. Mindfulness-based interventions are increasingly used to treat anxiety and panic disorders. Mindfulness is a technique that can help you ground your thoughts in the present. You can practice mindfulness by actively observing thoughts and sensations without reacting to them.

- Use relaxation techniques. Relaxation techniques include guided imagery, aromatherapy, and muscle relaxation. If you're experiencing symptoms of anxiety or a panic attack, try doing things that you find relaxing. Take a walk in a garden or park if available, close your eyes and apply the breathing technique above, take a bath, or use lavender, which has relaxing effects

**Buster #3 - Relaxation**

"Relaxation isn't only about peace of mind or enjoying a hobby.

Relaxation is a process that decreases the effects of stress on your mind and body."

Relaxation techniques can help you cope with everyday stresses from workplace to health related.

Whether your stress is out of control or you feel you can already control it, you can benefit from learning relaxation techniques. Learning basic relaxation techniques is easy. Relaxation techniques also are often free or low cost, pose little risk, and can be done nearly anywhere.

In today's busy world, relaxation techniques may not be a priority in your life, but not practising them means you will miss out on the health benefits.

The benefits of practising relaxation include:

- Slowing heart and breathing rate

- Lowering blood pressure

- Reducing muscle tension and chronic pain

- Improving concentration and mood

- Improving sleep quality and lowering fatigue

- Boosting confidence to handle problems

Relaxation techniques generally involve refocusing your attention on something calming and increasing awareness of your body, but to get even greater benefit, use relaxation techniques along with positive coping methods.

It doesn't matter which relaxation technique you choose. What matters is that you try to practice relaxation regularly to reap its benefits.

**The HACK: Consistency is key, and the more you practice, the more**

**effortless relaxation becomes.**

Why not try one of the following techniques?:

**Autogenic relaxation.** Using both visual imagery and body awareness to reduce stress, you repeat words or suggestions in your mind that help you relax and reduce muscle tension.

**Progressive muscle relaxation.** Focus on slowly tensing and then relaxing each muscle group. Start with your head and neck and work down to your toes. Tense your muscles for about five seconds and then relax for 30 seconds, and repeat.

**Visualisation.** Form mental images to take a visual journey to a peaceful, calming place or situation. Incorporate as many senses as you can, including smell, sight, sound and touch. Imagine relaxing at the ocean, and think about the smell of salt water, the sound of crashing waves and the warmth of the sun on your body.

Other relaxation techniques include:

*Reiki*
*Meditation*
*Tai chi or Qigong*
*Yoga*
*Aromatherapy*

All and any of these 'busters,' if you apply the HACK element, will work far more effectively than just the elements themselves. I know because I have trialed them many times and use them with my students regularly to great effect.

# PART NINE
## ABOUT THE AUTHOR

## *Laurence Nicholson*

**Laurence Nicholson is a Global-Award Winning 'Burnout Prevention Educator (Burnout Hacker)' the CEO and founder of 'burnout-hacker.com'**, as well as the CEO and Founder of the N Cubed Group, My Better Life Coaching, and Exec Mental Health Solutions, through which he works with both corporate clients and individuals, to improve and optimise mental health, cognitive performance and resilience, in order to realise measurable improvements in both business, and personal, productivity as well as decision making, but more importantly, understand how to prevent suffering the real trauma of burnout, and so protecting their families and lifestyles from its impacts.

He has spent over 35 years working around the world, across personal and corporate environments, as both a consultant and leader, and since experiencing 2 significant burnouts himself some 10 years ago, neuroscience, human psychology and behavioural patterns have become his passion, and he now uses his travelling to study wide and diverse behaviours, and investigate the 'how and why' of our brain's processes, and more importantly the impacts of stress and change on people, universally.

He also coaches others in how to educate people in Burnout Prevention, most recently in Tokyo, Japan just before the pandemic, with his Cognitive Masterclass. Part of his Burnout Prevention Educator Certification.

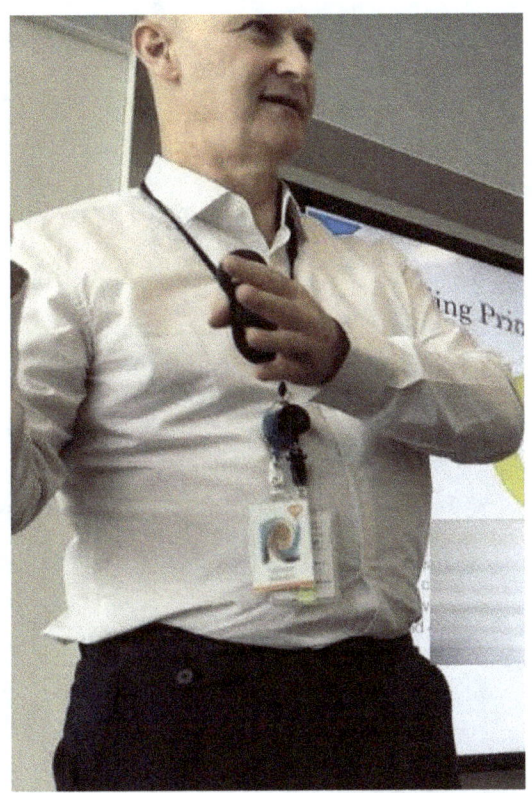

To stay updated with his courses, coaching and retreats, 'follow' on Facebook at 'https://www.facebook.com/burnout.hacks' or take out an exclusive membership for 'Burnout-Hackers' Private Group for regular content and articles, with ongoing group discussions by contacting Laurence at 'laurence@burnout-hacker.com'.

# Part Ten
## A Final Word...

## Reviews And Thanks...

Following a preview of this book given to a target group in 2020, I received many messages of support and personal experiences. Here are just a couple:

> "The emotional journey through Laurence's Burnout, made me more aware of our fragility and also provided explanations I had been missing for many of the signs I have personally experienced of possible onset of Burnout impacts. As a standalone read, this is invaluable, and I can only imagine the benefits his Cognitive Masterclass will bring to his students. I have already signed up!"
> - Jason, UK

> "WOW! I could feel his pain and loss acutely, as I read Laurence's story, and I am somewhat ashamed that I never thought about nor understood just how traumatic a real Burnout can be. The 'secret hacks' are great, and if this is just a 'taster' for the detail his Coaching goes into, I can see why his live workshops get booked up so far in advance! A must read for literally everyone!"
> - Sarah, UK

> "I missed Laurence's live sessions in Japan when he was here in 2018 and 2019, because they were fully booked! I am on the list for his first session when he returns. His story is

*saddening, and created many emotions in me as I have experienced a very much smaller burnout myself, but I celebrate the fact that it was the catalyst for his fantastic hacks, which I find invaluable! A fantastic source of knowledge!"*
     - Mika, Tokyo

My thanks go to everyone I met and who attended my courses, all of whom made me very welcome and made my whole experience on the trip one to cherish.


\*\*\*\*   END   \*\*\*\*